Sweat-Free Exercises for the Office

Also by Amanda Sterczyk

Balance Exercises for Fall Prevention

Balance 2.0:
Preventing Falls with Exercise

Your Job Is Killing You:
A User's Guide to Sneaking Exercise into Your Work Day

Balance and Your Body:
How Exercise Can Help You Avoid a Fall

Move More, Your Life Depends On It:
Practical Tips to Add More Movement to Your Day

I Can See Your Underwear:
My Journey Through the Fitness World

Sweat-Free Exercises for the Office

Amanda Sterczyk

Sterczyk, Amanda, author
    Your Job Is Killing You: A User's Guide to Sneaking Exercise into Your Work Day / Amanda Sterczyk.

Includes bibliographical references.
Issued in print and electronic formats.

ISBN 9798703891520

    1. Sedentary Work 2. Desk Bound 3. Exercise at Work 4. Stay Healthy at Work 5. Office

Cover image: Get Covers
Layout: Matthew Bin
Published by Kindle Direct Publishing

We are not tied to a desk or to a bench; we stay there only because we think we are tied.
— *Bolton Hall, 1854-1938*

CONTENTS

INTRODUCTION

Do you have a desk-based job? Are you a professional sitter? The knowledge-based economy means that many adults sit at their desks and in meetings for hours at a time every day. Productivity, profit, and professionalism lead people to remain seated at all times. But we're not in an airplane, and there is no turbulence. This physical inactivity is killing us.

Being sedentary for too long impacts your entire body—your brain feels sluggish, your joints hurt, your muscles stiffen, and your mood turns generally gloomy. I think we can all agree that it's difficult to be a happy, productive person when you feel like that.

My previous book for desk jockeys, _Your Job Is Killing You: A User's Guide to Sneaking Exercise Into Your Work Day_, was a self-help book, designed to help employees nudge themselves to sit less and move more during the work day. Although it was well-received, I still had people asking for an exercise manual. Specifically, they wanted sweat-free exercise options for sneaking a mini workout into their work day.

To date, I had only produced exercise guides for seniors—balance and strength bodyweight exercises that improved posture and flexibility in the process. When I mentioned that to an office worker, they told me, "That's probably all I could handle, because I feel so stiff and hunched over when I finally get up from my desk."

They're not alone. Physical inactivity is prematurely aging our mostly sedentary bodies when we sit at a desk all day. And that's how *Sweat-Free Exercises for the Office* was born. The exercises in this book don't require any special equipment or expensive exercise clothing. You can complete them in your work clothes and you won't even break a sweat—unless of course you want to, that is. If you tackle the exercises one at a time, whenever you have a free moment in the day, you'll enjoy a sweat-free experience. On the other hand, you may want to dedicate 30 minutes and flow from one exercise to the next, increasing the number of reps you do. In that case, might I suggest you slip into some workout clothes and keep a towel handy? Both options bring immediate benefits to your body and mind.

This book has seated and standing exercises. If you're stuck on a call and need to stay at your desk, you can add a little movement with some of the seated exercises. The standing exercises require a bit more space and, in some cases, include instructions for using a sturdy desk or wall. The appendix features a movement checklist to help you add some non-exercise, mini movement breaks to your work day. Our bodies need exercise and non-exercise activity, so the appendix is helpful supplement to the exercises.

CHAPTER ONE:
SITTING AND YOUR HEALTH

How Physically Active Are You?

Are you an active couch potato? Perhaps you're a weekend warrior? Even if you exercise on a regular basis, too much sitting during the rest of your waking hours can cause your body to resist the beneficial effects of that exercise. This is exactly what we're learning from new research into the impact of physical inactivity on our ability to benefit from moderate to vigorous physical activity.[i] It's almost as if your body goes into a slumber when you're sedentary, and the exercise isn't enough to wake it up and get it working properly.

Much has been written about the seemingly magical benefits of reversing the aging process with exercise.[ii] But that's not really an accurate portrayal of exercise and aging. In fact, active older adults are more like our ancestors. And sedentary younger adults—including those of middle age— are the ones who are prematurely aging themselves with physical inactivity.

That's why the World Health Organization has raised the alarm on physical inactivity, identifying it as the fourth leading risk factor for premature death, behind high blood pressure, tobacco use, and high blood sugar.[iii] The good news for people who are less physically active is that it doesn't take much to reduce the risk of death by sitting.[iv] In fact, one study showed that replacing just 30 minutes of daily sitting time with light physical activity resulted in a decrease in cancer, cardiovascular disease, and all-cause mortality. To me, that's another example of "a little goes a long way."

The activity our bodies crave and need can happen in minuscule increments. Indeed, a study in the *Journal of the American Heart Association* reported that physical activity that was accumulated in sporadic bouts throughout the day still reduced the risk of early death.[v] The total amount of daily physical activity is more important than how you accumulate that activity.

If you're already a frequent gym rat, keep it up. But make sure you're also adding movement throughout the rest of your day. And if you're not a gym user, take heart in the fact that you can still live a long and healthy life if you adopt a more active, less sedentary way of life. And that includes your time at the office. Is Sitting the New Smoking?

What's wrong with sitting for too long? When we sit for too long, our bones move out of alignment, and they stop doing their job. Our skeletons are designed to carry our body weight, but when the bones aren't aligned, the job falls instead to connective tissue like tendons and ligaments. This can lead to soft tissue injuries, pain, and discomfort. In addition, when we don't use our bones to hold our bodies in motion, they become weak. And when the bones of our spine start to compress, we suffer from disc damage and the associated pain.

The lack of movement from too much sitting also shortens our muscles, which means they stop working together properly. Some muscles, like our lower back and hips, get tight. Others, like our glutes and abs, become weak and/or overstretched. This muscular imbalance can cause back pain because our muscles can't hold our bones in proper alignment.

Further up the body, our shoulders rotate, our head hunches forward, and our upper spine looks more like a T than its natural C curve. This gives us a sore neck, shoulders, and upper back, and it makes it difficult to sit up straight. In turn, this imbalance of muscles—some tight, some weak, none functioning optimally—likewise impacts the range of motion in our joints, which translates to diminished balance and a heightened risk of falling.

Worried yet? That's not all. When our muscles don't function optimally, they stop helping our circulatory system pump blood to every nook and cranny in our bodies, reducing circulation. As a result, blood can pool in the feet and ankles because our muscles are not helping to pump that blood back up our bodies. Think swollen ankles, varicose veins, and blood clots.[vi] At the top of the house, our brains become fuzzy because of the reduced circulation of blood and oxygen. And I'm sure you can relate to what this means for work: difficulty concentrating on the task at hand.

Are You Aging or Just Physically

Inactive?

When you stand up, how long does it take you to go from sitting to standing? Do you feel stiffness in certain joints as you get up? Those moving parts, aka your joints, are seizing up from lack of lubrication. It's like glue drying: The moisture in your muscles and joints disappears. When you are stiff, you move more slowly until you can get your joints and muscles lubricated by moving. Then, you can increase the speed of your movements. Here's how it works.

Your circulatory system relies on your muscular system to move blood and oxygen to all the cells in your body. When you stop moving parts of your body for extended periods of time, cells dry up and die. It starts with muscle atrophy; that is, the cells in your muscles shrink from non-use.[vii] Your muscles shorten and pull the bones on either side of your joints closer together. Your muscles also become inflexible, which negatively impacts how much you can move—this is called the range of motion of your joints. That's why physically inactive individuals have a rounded back and stooped posture, not to mention a stiff and awkward gait that makes them appear older than they are.[viii]

Why do we consider stiff and slow movements to be a sign of aging? Because older adults who are less active behave and move the same way. When I work with sedentary office workers in their 40s and 50s, they have the same physical issues as individuals in their 70s and 80s.

When they get up and try to move around, these younger adults look older than they are.

Kind of scary, don't you think? Lack of physical movement is prematurely aging our society. So what's the solution? Move more. It's that simple. The exercises in this book will help you add some necessary movement and exercise to your work day.

What Does the Doctor Say?

Doctors are just as concerned about this wide-scale adoption of sedentary behaviour patterns. I recently interviewed Dr. Chris Raynor about this issue.[ix] Raynor is an orthopaedic surgeon and sports medicine specialist based in Ottawa. Here's what he had to say during our question and answer session.

Q: In the past, you've written about your experience as an orthopaedic surgeon, describing how many of your patients present with issues that could have been prevented with a daily dose of physical activity. Can you elaborate?

A: "In my practice, I see a lot of patients with various musculoskeletal complaints, many of which I feel can be remedied by regular doses of physical activity. It is important to note that studies now show that simply working out on a regular basis, although beneficial, does not counteract regular and prolonged sedentary activity. Therefore, it is necessary for us to re-evaluate the way we think about fitness, and how we incorporate it into our lives.

Studies also show that those people who are intermittently active throughout the day, generally measure higher on indices of health than do those who are mainly sedentary but who exercise regularly for one defined period of time. This suggests that it is more favourable for us as humans to incorporate activity throughout the day at multiple intervals, even if it's at a lower intensity, rather than exercise just once at a higher intensity."

Q: What type of advice do you give your patients, with regards to physical activity?

A: "I encourage my patients to implement easy movements and physical activities throughout the day in order to achieve this goal, and to keep them healthy and mobile over the long term. Of course, I suggest all the usual things like take the stairs, walk or bike to work or school, do walking meetings, find physical hobbies that you enjoy like hiking, gardening, dancing, etc. I also create challenges and physical literacy games that they can try. For example, I encourage most people -- especially those with lower extremity issues -- to do squat holds for a combined total of 10 minutes per day.[x] There are a few exceptions, but not many. Besides forcing them to get up from sitting on a regular basis, this is great for hip, knee, and ankle mobility, as well as lower limb and core strength. It is simple but effective, and in an attempt to hold them accountable, I test them on it when they see me in the office, so they know to practice. It seems to help—a lot."

Q: What type of reasons do you hear for people to NOT follow through on your advice for physical activity?

A: "There are a few who admit to NOT doing it. They say they don't have time, or it hurts too much. Or they say they did it for a week and didn't notice a difference, so they stopped. In response, I advise that it must become a habit. If they are having trouble with the initial suggestion, I tell them to start with a lower expectation and lower degree of difficulty, so if 10 minutes of squat hold every day is too much, they could try once a week for three minutes, or three times a week for five minutes—whatever they can manage. Instead of abandoning the goal altogether, they just need to make it easier. If it hurts too much to do a full-depth squat hold, I show them easier progressions: only going part way, and/or holding onto something for support. If they say they don't see a difference, I tell them that this is a long-term goal. There are solutions to every problem."

Q: Any final tips or words of advice?

A: "I also tell my patients that in terms of overall fitness, the little things make more of a difference than they think, and that they should take advantage of any opportunity to move around throughout the day—walk, stand, balance, reach, lift, carry, etc.—as much as possible. I tell them that you don't have to run 10 miles or lift weights for an hour all the time. It's about keeping joints lubricated and muscles supple, and keeping your blood sugar levels low, which is achieved by low to moderate activity at frequent and regular intervals."

So there you have it, straight from the doctor's office: add more mini-movement breaks throughout the day for optimal health. Before you begin the exercises, please take a moment to read the next chapter, which covers exercise setup and safety.

---

i   Alex Hutchison, "How your office job is affecting your metabolism," *The Globe and Mail*, March 22, 2019, https://www.theglobeandmail.com/life/health-and-fitness/article-how-your-office-job-is-affecting-your-metabolism/.

ii   Stephen Harridge & Norman Lazarus, "Can exercise reverse the ageing process?" *BBC News* (website), March 20, 2019, https://www.bbc.com/news/health-47331544.

iii   World Health Organization, *Global Health Risks: Mortality and Burden of Disease Attributable to Selected Major Risk* (Geneva: World Health Organization, 2009), http://www.who.int/healthinfo/global_burden_disease/GlobalHealthRisks_report_full.pdf.

iv   Erika Ress-Punia et al., "Mortality risk reductions for replacing sedentary time with physical activities," *American Journal of Preventive Medicine* 56, no. 5 (May 2019), 736-741, https://doi.org/10.1016/j.amepre.2018.12.006.

v   Pedro F. Saint-Maurice et al., "Moderate-to-Vigorous Physical Activity and All-Cause Mortality: Do Bouts Matter?" Journal of the American Heart Association (March 22, 2018), https://doi.org/10.1161/JAHA.117.007678.

vi   Berkowitz, The Health Hazards of Sitting.

vii   Miranda Esmonde-White, *Aging Backwards: 10 Years Younger, 10 Years Lighter, 30 Minutes A Day* (Toronto: Random House Canada, 2014), 37.

viii George Cranston, "Muscle Atrophy: Symptoms, Causes and Treatments," Health Guidance (blog), January 24, 2012, http://www.healthguidance.org/entry/14727/1/muscle-atrophy-symptoms-causes-and-treatments.html.

ix Online interview conducted with Dr. Chris Raynor via email, April & May 2019.

x A squat hold is an isometric exercise, which means that the muscles you will be working don't actually move during the exercise. You lower your body into a squat position and hold yourself in that position for as long as you can.

CHAPTER TWO:
EXERCISE SETUP

The Safety Talk

Before we proceed, let's talk about safety. As with other fitness texts, my book includes a disclaimer in the front: "The information in this book should not be used for diagnosis or treatment, or as a substitute for professional medical care. Before beginning any exercise program, consult your physician." That's not just legal jargon for the sake of it—it's important advice to heed because everyone's health is different.

But there's more: I want you to use your common sense. The exercises in this book are meant to help you, not hurt you. If something bothers you, STOP doing it. Always make sure you have something sturdy to hang onto—a counter, a wall, or a chair that won't slip.

These are exercises you can do in your workspace—be it a home or traditional office. As you start each exercise, focus on making slow, purposeful movements. If you feel dizzy, stop and sit down. If the feeling persists, consult your doctor.

Can we talk about feet now? I'm a barefoot soul - I much prefer to have my feet unencumbered by shoes and socks. But I know not everyone feels that way. And you may not feel comfortable with removing your shoes in the workplace. The exercises can be completed with or without footwear, EXCEPT if you are wearing high heels. I would advise against completing these exercises in high-heeled shoes.

Balance Definitions

As you work through the exercises, you may see some of the terms below. I've provided definitions, so you will understand the concepts.

Balance is a "sweet spot" between our base of support—typically our feet—and our centre of gravity—our weight distribution—while we're moving or standing still in an upright position.

Base of support: This refers to the area beneath you—whether you are standing or sitting—that makes contact with the surface that supports you. Reducing your base of support challenges your body's stability, as does changing your centre of gravity.

Centre of gravity: This refers to the point in your body around which your weight is evenly distributed. When you bend your knees, your centre of gravity is lowered.

What's the Speed Limit?

When you move on to the exercise section, you'll see that many of my instructions say things like, "slowly," or "with control." My intention is to have you focus on controlled movements that help to strengthen the muscles and increase mobility in the joints being targeted. Sometimes, we may want to rush moves—if, for example, we find them difficult and want to complete them faster. Or you may be trying to fit in a quick workout between meetings. But rushing the movement means you may actually be relying on movement, instead of muscle power. My recommendation is to slow it down and focus on the muscles needed to execute the exercise.

Please Keep Breathing

It's very important to remember to breathe as you complete the exercises. That's because holding your breath when you're exerting your body can place unnecessary strain on your heart. A helpful rule of thumb is to inhale and exhale for each step. For example: Inhale to complete step 1, exhale to complete step 2. Repeat. Depending on which part of an exercise sequence you find most difficult, you'll want to modify your breathing so that you're exhaling on the most strenuous portion. If you inhale during the most difficult part, you're more likely to hold your breath at the end of the inhalation.

Don't Forget to Warm Up

If you're wondering about warmups, let's chat about that now. The purpose of a warmup is to prepare your body for the exercises you are about to do, that is, the workout you're preparing to undertake. A warmup gets your blood pumping, gradually and safely increasing your heart rate and blood circulation. It loosens up stiff joints and delivers blood to the muscles you're about to use, preventing the risk of an injury.

Even if you're planning to tackle these exercises one at a time—that is, one exercise per break from work—your body will still benefit from warming up for at least two minutes. But don't worry, it doesn't have to be complicated. Here are three simple moves you can do to get warmed up and ready to exercise:

- One minute of marching on the spot,
- 30 seconds of shoulder rolls, and
- 30 seconds of arm swings.

Are you ready to begin? Then let's get started.

CHAPTER THREE: SEATED EXERCISES

Active Sitting

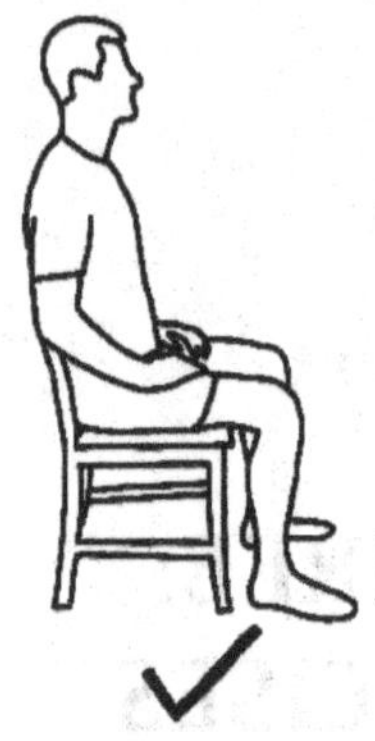
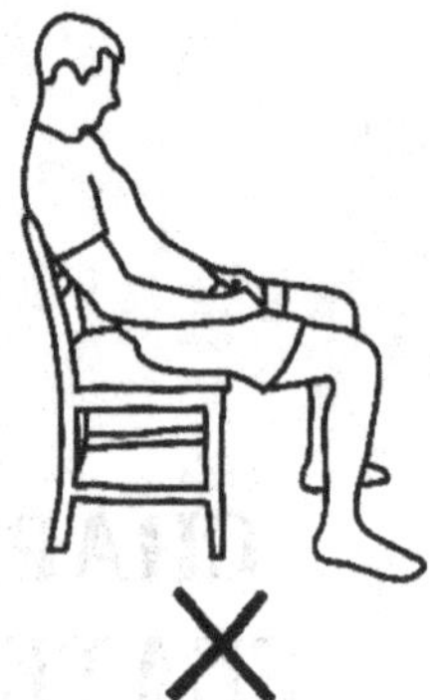

Active sitting helps us engage our muscles, strengthen our bones, and improve our posture. Instead of outsourcing the role of our muscles by slumping in our seats, we should sit tall.

To start: Begin by sitting in a chair that has a firm seat.

1. Shifting forward: Slide your bottom forward so you're not leaning back in the chair. Place both feet flat on the floor in front of you. If your legs are shorter and you can't touch the floor, you can place a large book or block on the floor to support your feet. Don't roll onto your tailbone. Imagine you have a tail and you want the tail behind you so you can wag it. Often, people roll backwards so they're resting on their tailbone instead of their sit bones—these are the

bony part of your bum, the lower edge of your pelvis.

2. Shoulder position: Drop your shoulders away from your ears. It should feel like you're letting them slide down your back.

3. Head position: Pull your head and neck back so your ears are sitting over your shoulders, not pushed forward. Your head is now positioned over your centre of gravity, which is allowing you to strengthen your bones by loading them. Feel your muscles and bones at work.

4. Aim for five minutes of active sitting every hour.

Visualize: A string is tied to the top of your head, pulling you up towards the ceiling.

Do you need to make it easier? Start with two minutes of active sitting.

Are you ready to make it harder? Try for 10 minutes of active sitting every hour.

Seated Joint Mobility

Our bodies are brilliant machines that are designed to move all day, every day. In our daily lives, we twist, we turn, we bend, we reach, and we lift. We use our bodies as a unit, and we expect to be able to move every which way without pain or having to worry about proper alignment.

If all of our muscles are strong and our joints are mobile, they're all fulfilling their intended roles and we operate like a finely tuned machine. If there's a muscular imbalance, bones get pulled closer together, causing joint pain and postural misalignment. Some people describe the joint immobility as "stiffness." Do you feel stiff in certain joints when you've been sitting for too long? Those moving parts, aka your joints, are seizing up from lack of lubrication. It's like glue drying: the moisture in your muscles and joints disappears. When you are stiff, you move more slowly until you can get your joints and muscles lubricated by moving. Then, you can increase the speed of your movements.

CARs—Controlled Articular Rotations—involve making s-l-o-w, controlled circles that increase mobility in your joints. Drawing these circles helps you feel less stiff and move more fluidly. The following joint mobility exercises can be completed even when you can't leave your desk. Think about all the smaller joints that you can move while you're sitting on a conference call or in a meeting. The key is to make slow and controlled movements. Many times, I see people drawing fast and sloppy circles. Fight the urge to get through the exercises as quickly as possible. Try to make the circular movements last for at least the number of seconds listed in the instructions.

Neck

To start: Sit comfortably in a chair.

1. Clockwise: Looking straight ahead, rotate your head in a clockwise direction for five seconds.
2. Counterclockwise: Switch directions and repeat as you count another five seconds.

Visualize: The movement should look as if you're drawing a circle with the tip of your nose.

Do you need to make it easier? Count fewer seconds to complete the joint rotations, or repeat the sequence fewer times. Take breaks and rest.

Are you ready to make it harder? Please don't try to make it harder. CARs are a feel-good movement designed to keep your joints mobile. We don't want to force them to work harder, just better!

Shoulders

To start: Sit comfortably in a chair.

1. Joint position: Relax your shoulders and keep your arms dropped at your side.
2. Forward: Slowly roll your shoulders forward, up, back, and down as you count to five.
3. Backward: Repeat in the opposite direction: pull them down, back, up, and forward as you count another five seconds.
4. Repeat: Repeat this sequence five to ten times.

Visualize: The movement should look as if your shoulders are a carpet that you are unrolling.

Do you need to make it easier? Count fewer seconds to complete the joint rotations, or repeat the sequence fewer times. Take breaks and rest.

Are you ready to make it harder? Please don't try to make it harder. CARs are a feel-good movement designed to keep your joints mobile. We don't want to force them to work harder, just better!

Elbows

To start: Sit comfortably in a chair.

1. Joint position: Lift your arms out to the side at a slight angle. Bend your elbows so that your hands are pointing towards the floor.
2. Clockwise: Slowly make circles by rotating your lower arm—below the elbow—clockwise for five seconds.
3. Counterclockwise: Repeat in the other direction for another five seconds.
4. Repeat: Repeat this sequence five to ten times. Lower your arms to your sides when you are finished.

Visualize: Your arms look like a scarecrow and the rest of your body is a tin man, so the only joint able to move in this position is your elbow. Your fingers are slowly drawing circles on the ground.

Do you need to make it easier? Count fewer seconds to complete the joint rotations, or repeat the sequence fewer times. Take breaks and rest.

Are you ready to make it harder? Please don't try to make it harder. CARs are a feel-good movement designed to keep your joints mobile. We don't want to force them to work harder, just better!

Wrists

To start: Sit comfortably in a chair.

1. Joint position: Lift your hands in front of you at chest height.
2. Clockwise: Slowly rotate both of your wrists in a clockwise direction while you count to ten.
3. Counterclockwise: Slowly rotate your wrists in the opposite direction while you count to ten again.
4. Repeat: Repeat this sequence five to ten times. Lower your hands to your sides when you are finished.

Visualize: Two pots of jam are being held in front of you and your hands are slowly stirring the thick spread.

Do you need to make it easier? Count fewer seconds to complete the joint rotations, or repeat the sequence fewer times. Take breaks and rest. Complete the movement as a lying down exercise.

Are you ready to make it harder? Please don't try to make it harder. CARs are a feel-good movement designed to keep your joints mobile. We don't want to force them to work harder, just better!

Fingers

To start: Sit comfortably in a chair.

1. Joint position: Lift your hands in front of you and spread out your fingers. You will work both hands at the same time.

2. Clockwise: Starting with your pinky fingers, slowly draw circles with each pinky finger in a clockwise direction for five seconds.

3. Counterclockwise: Repeat in the opposite direction for five more seconds.

4. Repeat: Repeat circles in both directions with each finger. So after you have finished with your pinky fingers, move on to your ring fingers, then your middle fingers, and your index fingers. When it's time to work your thumbs, slow down the circles even more. They have a bigger range of motion, so try to make circles with them for seven to eight seconds in each direction.

Visualize: Two pots of jam are being held in front of you and your fingers are slowly stirring the thick spread.

Do you need to make it easier? Count fewer seconds to complete the joint rotations, or repeat the sequence fewer times. Take breaks and rest. Complete the movement as a lying down exercise.

Are you ready to make it harder? We don't want to force the joints to work harder, just better!

Waist

To start: Sit on the front edge of a chair with your feet planted on the ground. This will give you clearance to circle towards the back without hitting the back of your chair.

1. Clockwise: Slowly rotate your upper body in a clockwise circle as you count to five.
2. Counterclockwise: Repeat in a counterclockwise circle for five more seconds.
3. Repeat: Repeat this sequence five to ten times.

Visualize: You are a puppet, and the strings attached to your waist are being moved to slowly lean you forwards and then back, in a circular pattern.

Do you need to make it easier? Count fewer seconds to complete the joint rotations, or repeat the sequence fewer times. Take breaks and rest.

Are you ready to make it harder? Please don't try to make it harder. CARs are a feel-good movement designed to keep your joints mobile. We don't want to force them to work harder, just better!

Ankles

To start: Sit comfortably in a chair.

1. Joint position: Lift your right foot off the ground and bend your knee.
2. Clockwise: Count to ten as you draw circles with your foot by rotating your ankle in a clockwise direction.
3. Counterclockwise: Count to ten as you draw circles in the opposite direction.
4. Repeat: Repeat this sequence five to ten times, then lower your right foot to the ground.
5. Other ankle: Lift your left foot off the ground and repeat the entire sequence in both directions, then lower your left foot to the ground.
6. You can even try wiggling your toes a little. These aren't rotations, just an additional feel-good movement.

Visualize: Your foot is a pencil and you are using it to slowly draw circles on the ground.

Do you need to make it easier? Count fewer seconds to complete the joint rotations, or repeat the sequence fewer times. Take breaks and rest. Complete the movement as a lying down exercise.

Are you ready to make it harder? We don't want to force the joints to work harder, just better!

Seated Clock Toe Taps

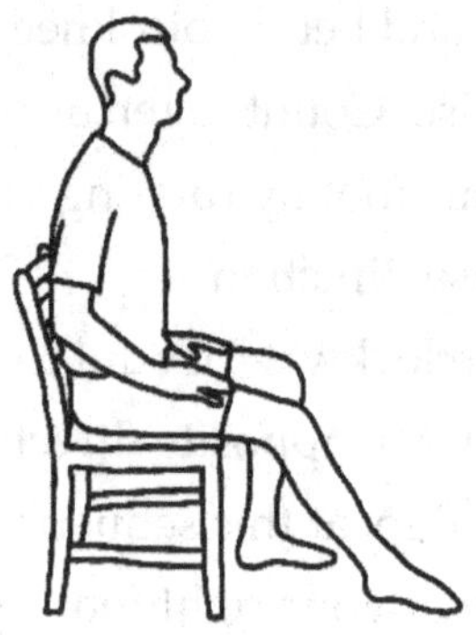

Clock toe taps as a seated exercise focus on hip mobility, as you straighten and bend your leg, rotating it in the hip socket.

To start: Sit on the edge of a sturdy chair. Make sure there are no obstacles in a semi-circle in front of you.

1. Twelve o'clock: Reach your right foot forward with a straight leg and gently tap your big toe at the 12 o'clock position, then return it to the ground beside your left foot.
2. Moving around the clock: Continue tapping your toe around the imaginary clock, always returning to the centre between each "hour" and placing your foot on the ground before continuing to the next "hour."
3. At the three o'clock position, repeat in the opposite direction, returning to 12 o'clock.

4. Switch legs: Repeat the toe taps with your left foot, beginning at 12 o'clock and working backwards from 11 o'clock down to nine o'clock. Repeat in the opposite direction, returning to 12 o'clock.

5. Try to do this exercise three times on each side.

Visualize: Imagine that there's a clock face on the floor and you're sitting in the middle of it. The goal is to tap each hour on the clock from 12 o'clock all the way to three o'clock/nine o'clock, and then repeat the toe taps in the opposite direction back to 12 o'clock.

Do you need to make it easier? If a particular position feels too difficult or uncomfortable, don't reach as far. Instead of tapping the toe on the ground, just lift the leg in that direction and return it to the centre, beside your other foot. Start by doing the exercises once on each leg, and gradually work your way up to three repetitions.

Are you ready to make it harder? Repeat this exercise as a standing exercise.

Double Gas Pedal

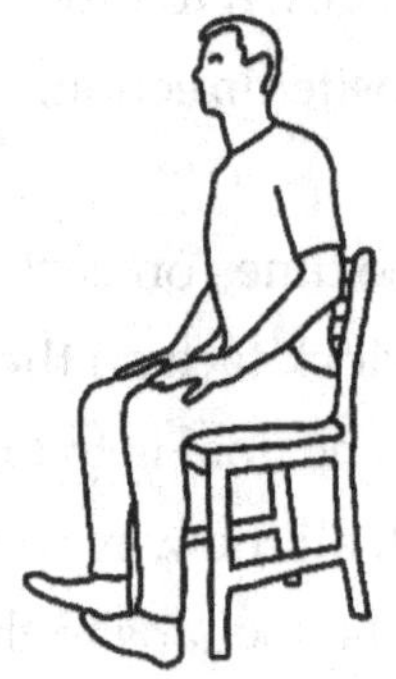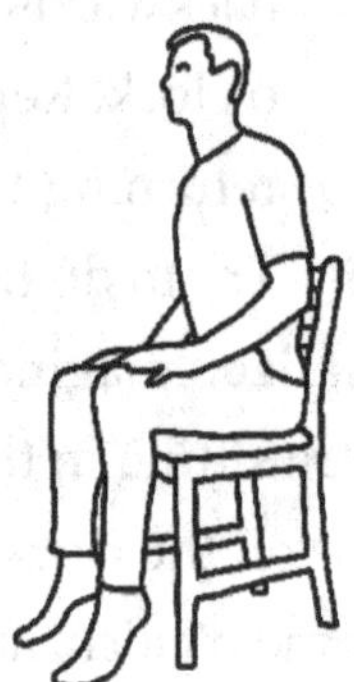

The gas pedal sequence will loosen up stiff ankles and strengthen the muscles in your calves and shins, thereby making walking easier and more fluid. Sitting at the front of the chair, rather than relying on the chair back for support, will further strengthen your core (aka your abdominal muscles). This exercise can be done wearing shoes or with bare feet.

To start: Sit tall in a chair, with both feet planted flat on the floor, hip-width apart. Look straight ahead and keep your body tall throughout the sequence.

1. Moving both feet at the same time, lift your toes off the floor.
2. Lower the toes to the starting position.
3. Lift both heels off the floor.
4. Lower the heels to the starting position.

Repeat steps 1 to 4 at least eight to 10 times.

Visualize: Your feet are a seesaw, moving up and down in a controlled fashion.

Do you need to make it easier? Focus on one foot at a time, then switch to the other foot.

Are you ready to make it harder? Stand up to increase the balance difficulty of the movement. Hang on to the back of your chair for support, and follow steps 1 to 4 standing.

Heel Slides

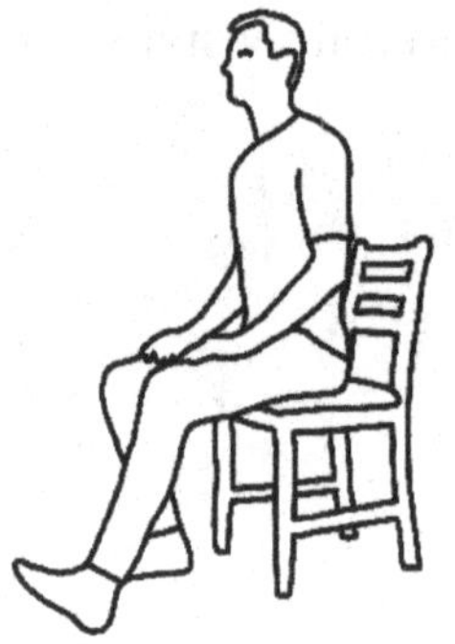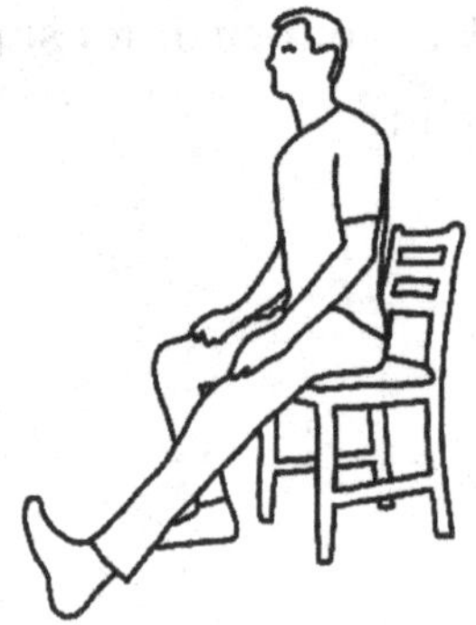

Heel slides work the muscles up the back of the leg, increasing lower limb strength and improving your walking stride. Sitting at the front of the chair, instead of relying on the chair back to hold your body upright, will further strengthen your core (aka your abdominal muscles). This exercise is best performed while wearing socks to allow your foot to slide more freely.

To start: Sit tall in a chair, with both feet planted flat on the floor, hip-width apart. Look straight ahead and keep your body tall throughout the sequence.

1. Straighten your right leg and flex your right foot, so your heel remains in contact with the ground, but your toes are pointing up towards the ceiling.
2. Squeeze your glute muscles and the back of your thigh, using these muscles to drag your

right heel back towards the chair while it remains in contact with the floor.

3. Reverse the movement and slide your heel away from you, straightening your right knee until you reach the starting position.

4. Perform 10–12 repetitions on the right side.

5. Repeat steps 1 to 4 with the left foot.

Visualize: Imagine driving a car with no hand break and you are on a hill, slide the leg out to push down on the brake pedal (squeeze your flute muscles to hold it there). Then, release the brake slowly as you slide your heel back towards the chair.

Do you need to make it easier? Stay closer to the chair (don't straighten your leg completely).

Are you ready to make it harder? Slide both heels out and back at the same time.

Torso Twists

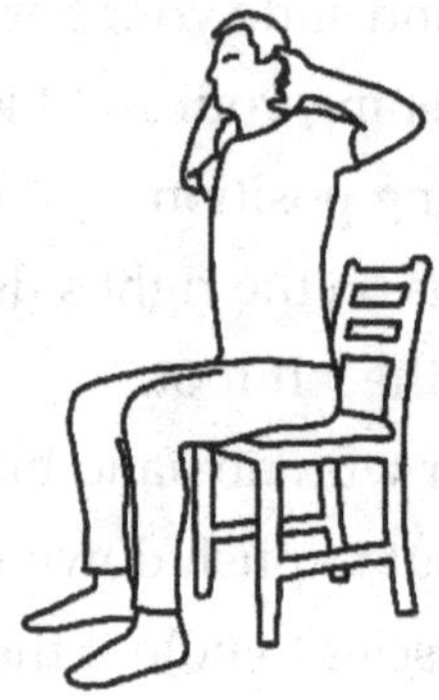 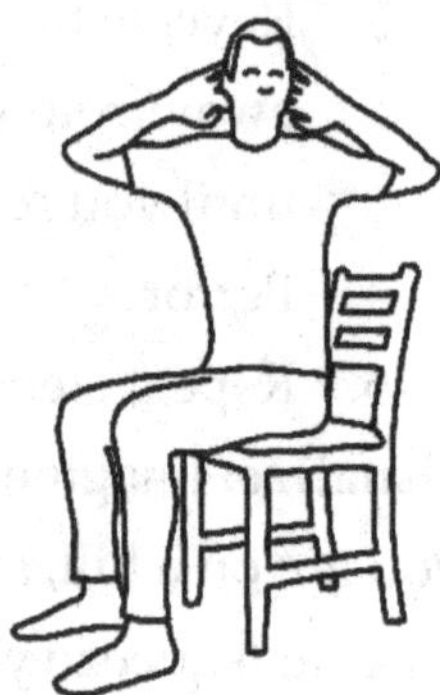

Torso twists work the abdominal muscles on the sides of your body, strengthening your core and improving the mobility of your spine. Both of these are important for maintaining good balance during functional activities, like twisting and turning as you empty your dishwasher or getting out of your car.

To start: Sit tall on a chair with your feet flat on the ground about hip-width apart. Make sure you don't lean back in the chair. Place your hands lightly behind your head, with your elbows bent and pointing out towards the sides of the room.

1. Slowly rotate your torso to the left as far as you comfortably can, keeping the rest of your body still, i.e. your bum doesn't move on the chair.
2. Rotate back to the starting position in the middle.

3. Continue rotating to the right side as far as you comfortably can, keeping the rest of your body still.

4. Rotate back to the starting position in the middle.

5. Repeat steps 1 to 4 at least eight to 10 times.

Visualize: Your body from your hips up to the top of your head is a key, turning as a solid unit back and forth in a lock.

Do you need to make it easier? Cross your arms in front of your chest to complete the sequence with a lower centre of gravity.

Are you ready to make it harder? Complete the torso twists while standing.

Reverse Sit-ups

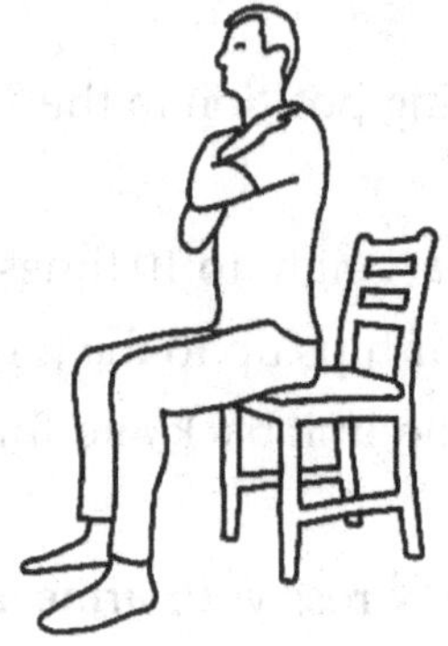 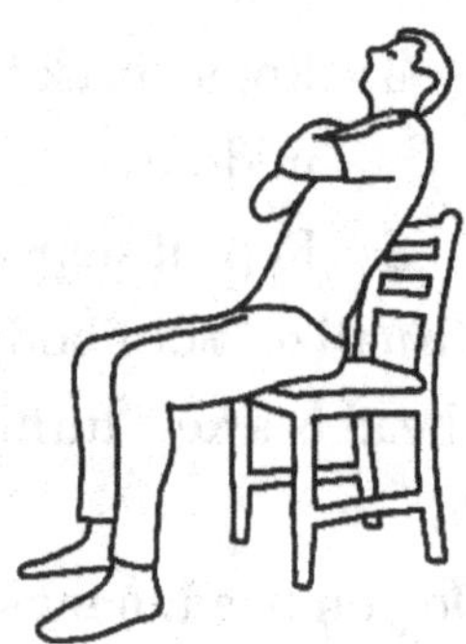

While everyone loves to hate sit-ups and other abdominal exercises, that's because they're targeting a part of our bodies that we often neglect. In addition to improving our core strength, sit-ups allow us to have better balance and stability, and improved posture. They also reduce the risk of back pain and injury.

To start: Sit tall on the edge of a chair with both feet planted flat on the floor, hip-width apart. Look straight ahead and cross your arms over your chest, with each hand touching the opposite shoulder.

1. Slowly lean back, moving your torso as a solid unit towards the back of your chair. Stop before your shoulder blades touch the chair.
2. Pull your body forward in a smooth motion, returning yourself to the upright starting position.
3. Repeat steps 1 and 2 at least eight to 10 times.

Tighten your stomach as if you're about to be tickled. Maintain that level of stiffness throughout the sequence.

Do you need to make it easier? Hook your hands on the sides of the chair, and follow steps 1 and 2.

Are you ready to make it harder? Bring your hands up beside your head, palms facing forward, elbows bent, with your fingertips touching your temples. Keep your hands in this position and follow steps 1 and 2.

Side to Side Arm Reaches

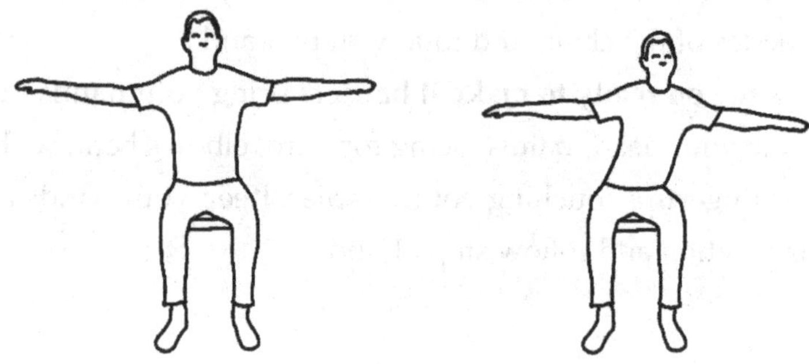

Side-to-side arm reaches work the abdominal muscles on the sides of your body, strengthening your core and improving the mobility of your spine.

To start: Sit tall on the edge of a chair, with both feet planted flat on the floor, hip-width apart. Look straight ahead. Lift your arms out to the side at shoulder height, with your elbows straightened.

1. Keeping your bum and hips planted on the chair, slowly lean your torso towards your left side, as if you're trying to touch something at shoulder height with your left hand. Don't tip your hand towards the floor.
2. Return to the centre, with your torso forming a straight line towards the ceiling.
3. Repeat the movement towards your right side.
4. Return to the centre starting position.
5. Follow steps 1 to 4 at least eight to 10 times.

Visualize: Your torso is bound by a metal cage, and your arms are the ropes in an evenly-matched tug of war.

Do you need to make it easier? Hook your hands on the sides of the chair, and follow steps 1 to 4.

Are you ready to make it harder? Follow steps 1 to 4, reaching even farther out to each side.

Seated Overhead Arm Raises

Ceiling reaches, even when completed whilst seated, improve our posture, strengthening both our muscles and our bones, helping us to stand and walk in a more upright position (as opposed to being hunched over). When we stand straighter, our muscles and bones are completing their intended role—to support our frame.

To start: Sit comfortably in a chair.

1. Lift your right arm above your head, straightening the elbow and maintaining a tall posture.
2. Lower your right arm to the starting position.
3. Lift your left arm above your head, straightening the elbow and maintaining a tall posture.
4. Lower your left arm to the starting position.
5. Continue alternating arm reaches until you have completed 10 on each side.

Visualize: You are a puppet, and the string holding up your head and torso is taut and unmoving, while the strings on your wrists alternately lift your arms upwards.

Do you need to make it easier? Focus on lifting your arm as high as possible, keep the elbow bent as needed.

Are you ready to make it harder? Repeat it as a standing exercise.

Seated Side Bends

Side bends work the muscles along the sides of your torso, helping to increase your upper body strength and maintain an upright posture.

To start: Sit comfortably in a chair.

1. Place your arms at your sides, fingertips facing down towards the floor.
2. At your waist, lean to your right side with your fingertips reaching towards the floor.
3. Move back to your starting position.
4. Continue bending to the right and up again five to 10 times.
5. Follow steps 1 to 4 on the left side.

Visualize: You're a teapot wedged between two sheets of glass, tipping over from the waist without leaning forward or back.

Do you need to make it easier? Start with 3 to 5 repetitions. Take frequent breaks and rest.

Are you ready to make it harder? Repeat it as a standing exercise.

Seated High March

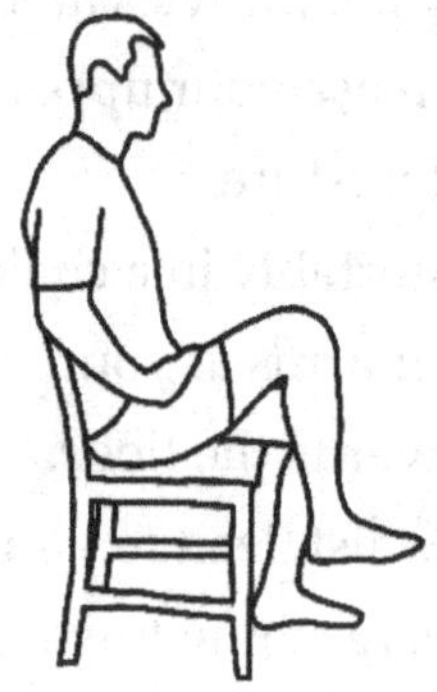

The seated high march is a strength exercise that creates stability on both sides of the body. You are working on your core stability, which helps with balance. Strong muscles and bones allow us to lift our legs and feet over obstacles, and avoid shuffling when walking, which can lead to falls.

To start: Sit on a chair with your feet flat on the ground and your bum close to the edge of the chair. Try to sit as tall as you can.

1. Lift: Lift one knee up as high as you can and hold it up for three to five seconds.
2. Lower: Use control to lower the leg to the starting position. (Don't use gravity!)
3. Repeat: Repeat Steps 1 and 2 on the other leg.
4. Aim for ten marches, alternating sides with each repetition.

Visualize: Your torso, from just above your hips right up to the top of your head, is frozen in a solid block of ice, and you can only move your legs up and down.

Do you need to make it easier? Start with as many as you can, and work your way up to ten. Take a break between each repetition.

Are you ready to make it harder? Repeat it as a standing exercise.

CHAPTER FOUR:
STANDING EXERCISES

Active Standing

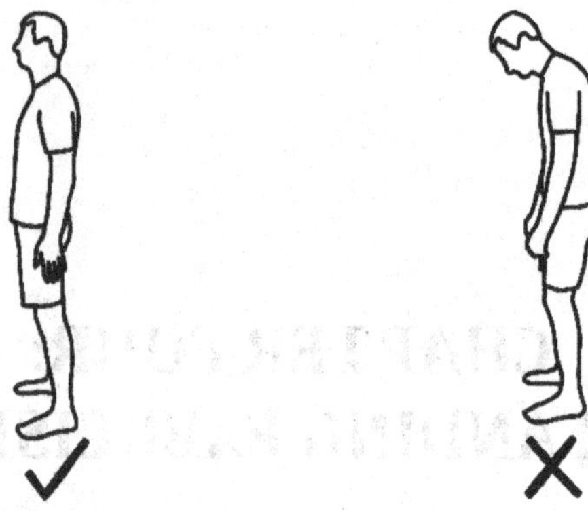

Active standing allows us to align our bones while strengthening our muscles and bones in the process. Active standing should feel like work. Your muscles are working together to hold you upright. This is a more effective way to stand, instead of dropping into your heels and hips. Resist the pull of gravity!

For this exercise, you can remove your shoes if you're willing to be bare foot.

To start: Stand up.

- Foot position: Imagine a triangle under each foot. Instead of sinking backwards onto your heels and dropping into your hips, engage your entire foot by transferring more weight forward and across the width of your foot. Your toes and heels on both feet should be pointing forwards, not turned in or out.

- Arm position: Allow your arms to hang smoothly at the sides of your body, not behind or in front of your torso. Your palms should be touching your thighs, not facing backwards.
- Shoulder position: Drop your shoulders away from your ears. It should feel like you're letting them slide down your back.
- Head position: Pull your head and neck back so your ears are sitting over your shoulders, not pushed forward. Your head is now positioned over your centre of gravity, which is allowing you to strengthen your bones by loading them. Feel your muscles and bones at work. Aim for five minutes of active standing every hour.

Visualize: A string is tied to the top of your head, pulling you up towards the ceiling.

Do you need to make it easier? Start with two minutes of active standing.

Are you ready to make it harder? Try for 10 minutes of active standing every hour.

Clock Toe Taps

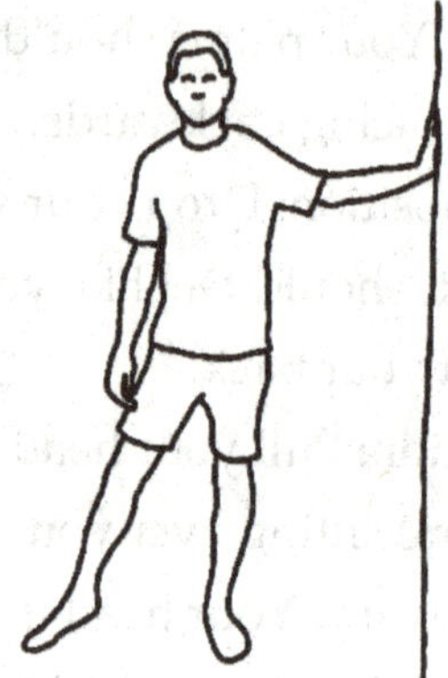

Clock toe taps improve your balance and hip mobility. Your standing leg is getting stronger, while your working leg is increasing the range of motion of your hip.

To start: Stand near a desk, wall, or sturdy chair, and hang on with your left hand. You will be working the right leg first, so make sure there are no obstacles in a semi-circle near your right leg.

- Twelve o'clock: Reach your right foot forward with a straight leg and gently tap your big toe at the 12 o'clock position, then return it to the ground beside your left foot. With your weight on your standing leg, gently but quickly tap your toe on the ground.
- Moving around the clock: Continue tapping your toe around the imaginary clock, always returning to the centre between each "hour" and placing your foot on the ground before continuing to the next "hour." Repeat in the opposite direction, returning to 12 o'clock.

- Switch legs: Once you have finished the exercise with your right leg, turn around and hold on to your support with your right hand.
- Repeat: Repeat the toe taps with your left foot, beginning at 12 o'clock and working backwards from 11 o'clock down to six o'clock. Repeat in the opposite direction, returning to 12 o'clock.
- Try to do this exercise three times on each leg.

Visualize: Imagine that there's a clock face on the floor and you're standing in the middle of it. The goal is to tap each hour on the clock from 12 o'clock all the way to six o'clock, and then repeat the toe taps in the opposite direction back to 12 o'clock.

Do you need to make it easier? If a particular position feels too difficult or uncomfortable, don't reach as far. Instead of tapping the toe on the ground, just lift the leg in that direction and return it to the centre, beside your standing foot. Sit on the edge of a sturdy chair and perform the toe taps from 12 o'clock to three o'clock on the right leg, and from 12 o'clock to nine o'clock on the left leg. Start by doing the exercises once on each leg, and gradually work your way up to three repetitions.

Are you ready to make it harder? If you feel strong and stable enough, complete the clock toe taps without holding on to your support.

Dynamic Walking

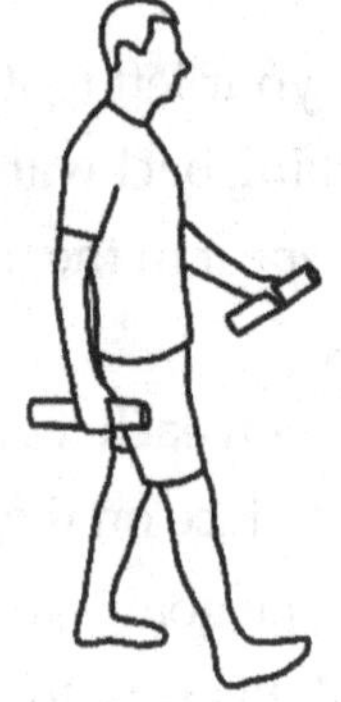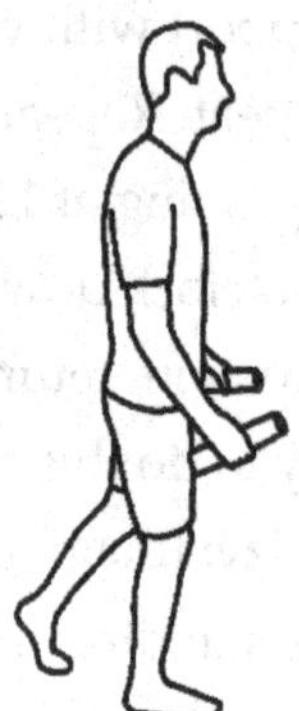

Walking is the ultimate dynamic balance challenge because you constantly shift your centre of gravity and base of support. Before you begin this exercise, make sure the surrounding area is clear of obstacles. Hallways are a great place to practice walking because the walls are close to you in case you need to steady yourself, and hallways are typically already clear spaces for moving about. If you are comfortable practicing outside, you can walk further. If you're staying indoors, make space to walk ten to 12 steps at minimum.

Equipment needed: Two empty paper towel tubes or pieces of paper rolled up and taped as tubes. Holding the tubes will keep your shoulders down and back, instead of rounded forward. This is a better posture for walking.

- Tubes: Hold a tube in each hand, with your hands at hip height. One open end of the tube should face forward while the other open end faces backward. The tubes will help you keep your shoulders rotated correctly. If you feel the open end of the tube touching your leg, you've rounded your shoulders and the tubes are no longer pointing forward and back.

- Shoulders: Drop your shoulders away from your ears as you maintain an upright posture. Imagine you're trying to slip your shoulder blades into your back pockets.

- These two steps will ensure that you're aligning your bones before you begin walking.

- Walk: To begin walking, lift one foot and bring it forward. As you lower it to the ground, use the entire foot. Plant your heel first, roll forward on to your foot, then push off the ball of your foot and big toe as you lift the other foot. This rolling movement helps propel you forward, using your leg muscles. What many people do, however, is swing their leg instead of pushing off the big toe. This movement weakens the muscles, which makes it difficult to lift that big toe up enough to clear the ground. Involving your entire body in the practice of walking properly will improve your balance and posture.

- Arms: Engage your arms as a counterbalance. That means that when your left foot is forward, your right arm should move forward. When your right foot is forward, your left arm should move forward.

Do you need to make it easier? Skip the first two steps and go straight to Step 3, holding on to the wall with one hand as you practice planting your heel, rolling through your foot, then pushing off the front of your foot. You can also try using walking poles or some other stability device to increase your base of support and help hold you upright.

Are you ready to make it harder? Replace the paper towel tubes with light hand weights, and try to increase your walking speed.

Joint Mobility

Our bodies are brilliant machines that are designed to move all day, every day. In our daily lives, we twist, we turn, we bend, we reach, and we lift. We use our bodies as a unit, and we expect to be able to move every which way without pain or having to worry about proper alignment.

If all of our muscles are strong and our joints are mobile, they're all fulfilling their intended roles and we operate like a finely tuned machine. If there's a muscular imbalance, bones get pulled closer together, causing joint pain and postural misalignment. Some people describe the joint immobility as "stiffness." Do you feel stiff in certain joints when you've been sitting for too long? Those moving parts, aka your joints, are seizing up from lack of lubrication. It's like glue drying: the moisture in your muscles and joints disappears. When you are stiff, you move more slowly until you can get your joints and muscles lubricated by moving. Then, you can increase the speed of your movements.

CARs—Controlled Articular Rotations—involve making s-l-o-w, controlled circles that increase mobility in your joints. Drawing these circles helps you feel less stiff and move more fluidly. The following joint mobility exercises can be completed from a standing position. The key is to make slow and controlled movements. Many times, I see people drawing fast and sloppy circles. Fight the urge to get through the exercises as quickly as possible. Try to make the circular movements last for at least the number of seconds listed in the instructions.

Waist

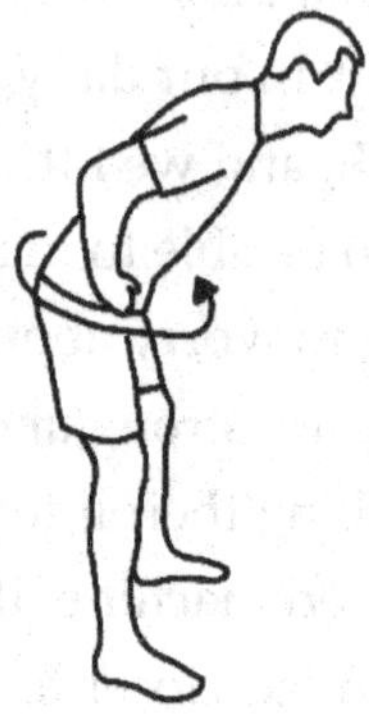

To start: Keep your feet at hip's width. You can put your hands on your hips or stretch them out to the sides before you begin.

1. Clockwise: Slowly rotate your upper body in a clockwise circle as you count to five.
2. Counterclockwise: Repeat in a counterclockwise circle for five more seconds.
3. Repeat: Repeat this sequence five to ten times.

Visualize: You are a puppet, and the strings attached to your waist are being moved to slowly lean you forwards and then back, in a circular pattern.

Do you need to make it easier? Count fewer seconds to complete the joint rotations, or repeat the sequence fewer times. Take breaks and sit down for a rest. Complete the movement as a seated exercise.

Are you ready to make it harder? We don't want to force the joints to work harder, just better!

Hips

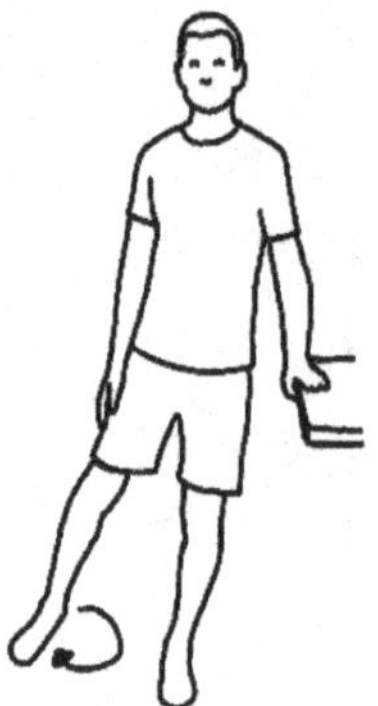

To start: Stand beside a desk, wall, or sturdy chair. Hang on for support.

1. Joint position: Lift your right foot off the ground while holding on to your support with your left hand. You can lean on your support to do these—that way, your moving foot won't hit the ground.

2. Clockwise: Count to ten as you slowly draw circles with your leg. The movement should come from your hip socket so that you are rotating your whole leg, with your leg straight. If you find it too difficult to make circles with your leg straight, try bending your knee.

3. Counterclockwise: Count to ten again as you draw circles with your leg in the opposite direction.

4. Repeat: Repeat this sequence five to ten times, then lower your right foot to the ground.

5. Other hip: Change your body position so that you can hang on to your support with your right hand. Lift your left foot off the ground and repeat the entire sequence. Lower your left foot to the ground.

Visualize: Your leg is a pencil and you are drawing circles on the ground.

Do you need to make it easier? Count fewer seconds to complete the joint rotations, or repeat the sequence fewer times. Take breaks and sit down for a rest.

Are you ready to make it harder? Please don't try to make it harder. CARs are a feel-good movement designed to keep your joints mobile. We don't want to force them to work harder, just better!

Knees

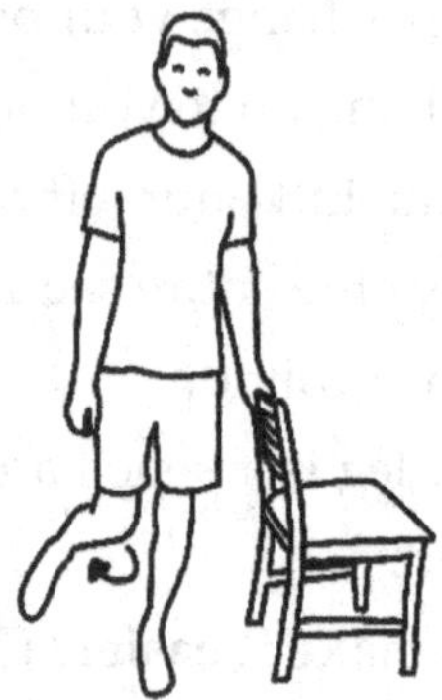

To start: Stand beside a desk, wall, or sturdy chair. Hang on for support.

1. Joint position: Lift your right foot off the ground and bend the knee.
2. Clockwise: Count to ten as you draw circles using the lower part of your right leg—below the knee—in a clockwise direction.
3. Counterclockwise: Count to ten as you draw circles in the opposite direction.
4. Repeat: Repeat this sequence five to ten times, then lower your right foot to the ground.
5. Other knee: Lift your left foot off the ground and repeat the entire sequence. Lower your left foot to the ground.

Visualize: Your body is a tin man, so the only joint able to move in this position is your knee. Your lower leg is slowly drawing circles on the ground.

Do you need to make it easier? Count fewer seconds to complete the joint rotations, or repeat the sequence fewer times. Take breaks and sit down for a rest. Complete the movement as a seated exercise.

Are you ready to make it harder? Please don't try to make it harder. CARs are a feel-good movement designed to keep your joints mobile. We don't want to force them to work harder, just better!

Overhead Arm Raises

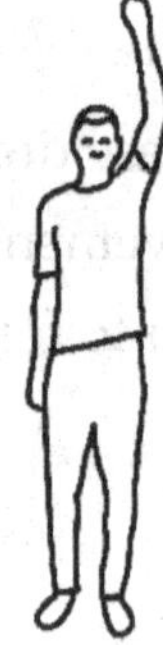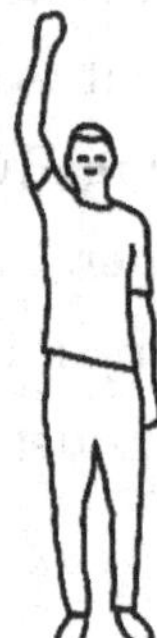

Our torso can help keep us upright for exercises like overhead arm reaches. This improves our posture, strengthening both our muscles and our bones. When we stand straighter, it is easier to walk with a straighter frame and see where we are going, thus reducing the likelihood of a momentum-based fall. These reaches will help you achieve that goal and keep you from toppling forward when you're walking.

To start: Stand tall with your feet facing forward, hip-width apart, with your arms hanging at your sides.

1. Lift your right arm above your head, straightening the elbow and maintaining a tall posture.
2. Lower your right arm to the starting position.
3. Lift your left arm above your head, straightening the elbow and maintaining a tall posture.
4. Lower your left arm to the starting position.

Continue alternating arm reaches until you have completed 10 on each side.

Visualize: You are a puppet, and the string holding up your head and torso is taut and unmoving, while the strings on your wrists alternately lift your arms upwards.

Do you need to make it easier? You can sit in a chair to complete the arm reaches.

Are you ready to make it harder? Try balancing on one foot to increase the difficulty of the arm reaches.

Standing Bird Dog

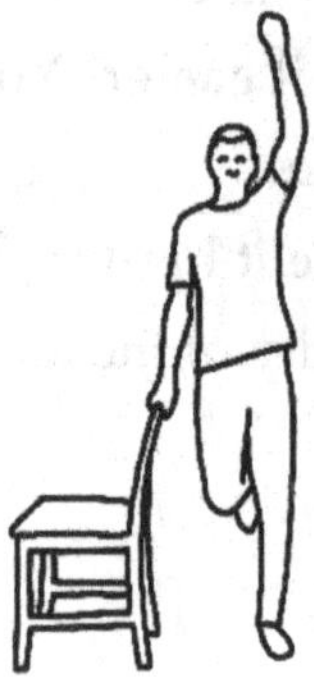

The bird dog exercise helps improve your posture by strengthening the muscles in your torso. It will increase your stability and coordination as you work on your balance.

To start: Stand beside a wall, desk, or sturdy chair. Hang on to your steady surface with your left hand.

1. Reach towards the ceiling with your right hand, making your arm as straight as possible above your head.

2. Lift the right leg off the ground. You can bend this leg at the knee to avoid leaning away from your support.

3. Hold this position—one arm up, one leg up—for as long as you can, up to 30 seconds. You may feel your body swaying a bit as you balance on one leg. Maintain a firm grip on your support to remain stable. Lower your foot to the ground if you're feeling too unsteady.

4. Return to the starting position: Lower your right leg and right arm.

5. Turn around to face the opposite direction and hold your support with your right hand.

Follow steps 1 to 4 with your left arm and leg.

Visualize: Your arm is the nose of a pointer dog, and your body is a stiff board from your outstretched fingers, down your arm, across your torso, through your balancing leg into the foot on the ground.

Four modifications are listed below. The first two will make it easier, while the second two increase the challenge of the exercise.

Do you need to make it easier? Instead of reaching your arm above your head, lift it away from your body—to the side or in front—at shoulder height. Or, instead of lifting your foot completely off the ground, employ the "kickstand" position: turn your toes away from your body, slide that foot towards your opposite ankle as you lift it off the ground, keeping your big toe on the ground for stability. The sole of this foot rests against the inside of your opposite leg at ankle height.

Are you ready to make it harder? Try the balance exercise without holding on to your support. Or, take it to the floor: Begin on your hands and knees, stretching an opposite arm and leg away from your centre.

Wall Pushup

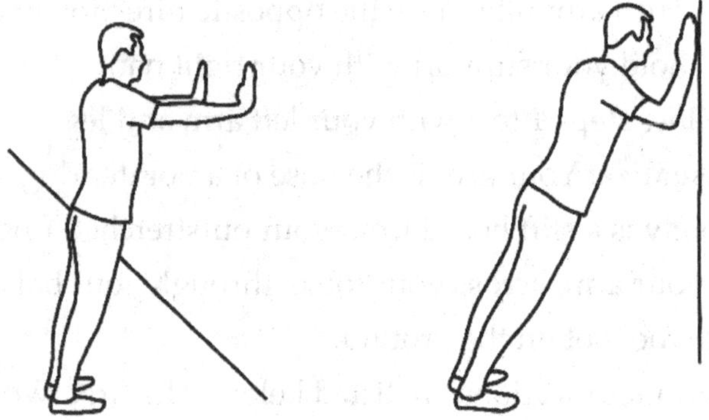

Push-ups are an effective exercise to build upper body strength. Your chest, shoulders, back, and arms all work together to move you with control. Your abdominal muscles also play a role in maintaining a stiff torso and preventing you from arching your back, thereby strengthening your entire core.

To start: To avoid slipping, do this exercise in shoes or bare feet. Stand facing a blank wall or closed door, with your feet hip-width apart. Your distance from the surface will depend on the length of your arms, so you may need to shift your feet forward or back before you begin.

1. Place your open palms against the door/wall, directly in front of your shoulders. Relax your shoulders down away from your ears, and squeeze your stomach muscles.
2. Check your elbows, they should be almost straight (not locked) in the starting position.

3. Slowly bend your elbows to bring your nose closer to the wall or door.
4. Straighten your arms to return to the starting position.
5. Repeat steps 3 and 4 at least five to 10 times.

Visualize: Your body from your shoulders down to your ankles is a solid board, that moves as a single unit.

Four modifications are listed below: The first two will make it easier, while the second two increase the challenge of the exercise.

Do you need to make it easier? Walk your feet forward, and begin with a bigger bend in your elbow. If this is still too difficult, sit on a chair with your feet flat on the ground and your bum close to the edge of the chair. Follow steps 1 to 5 from a seated position.

Are you ready to make it harder? Walk your feet further away so that you're leaning at a sharper angle. Follow steps 1 to 5. For an added challenge, lift one foot off the ground. Perform five wall push-ups on one foot. Switch to the other foot and repeat.

Desk Knee Lifts

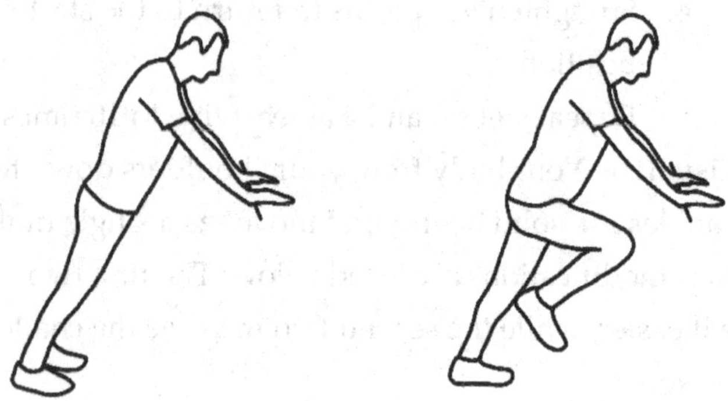

Also known as Mountain Climbers, desk knee lifts are a full-body exercise that work your legs, core, and upper body. They also qualify as a cardio exercise, as they help to elevate your heart rate. Performed against a sturdy desk, the angle will be less difficult than starting on the floor, which is described below as a modification to make the exercise more challenging.

To start: Place your hands on the edge of the counter, and walk your feet backward until your body is leaning at a 45-degree angle.

1. Pull your right knee to your chest as close as you can.
2. Lower your right foot back to the ground.
3. Pull your left knee to your chest, as close as you can.
4. Lower your left foot back to the ground.

Repeat steps 1 to 4 up to 10 times.

Visualize: Your body from your wrists, through your shoulders to your hips is a stiff, unmoving upside-down check mark. Keep your shoulders down and your stomach tense, moving only from your knees.

Four modifications are listed below: The first two will make it easier, while the second two increase the challenge of the exercise.

Do you need to make it easier? Bring your feet closer to the desk to decrease the lean of your body. Follow steps 1 to 4 in this position. If this angle is still too demanding, use a wall instead, placing your palms against the wall directly in front of your shoulders. Follow steps 1 to 4 in this position.

Are you ready to make it harder? Try to increase the speed at which you alternate pulling your knees to your chest. Want to make it even more challenging? Instead of leaning against a desk, complete this exercise on the floor. Begin in a plank position, holding yourself on your hands and toes. Line up your hands under your shoulders, with your legs extended behind you. Follow steps 1 to 4 in this position.

Heel-Toe Walk

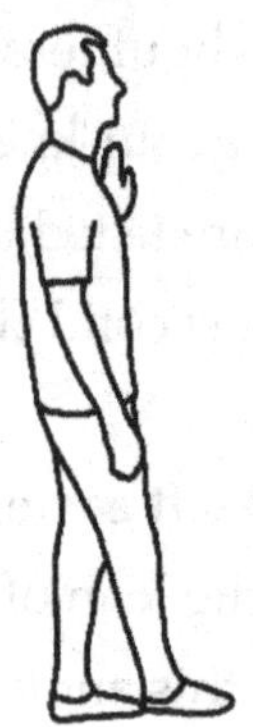

Heel-toe walking is a dynamic balance exercise that requires you to constantly shift your centre of gravity over a narrow base of support.

To start: Before you begin this exercise, make sure the surrounding area is clear of obstacles. Hallways are a great place to practice walking because the walls are close to you, in case you need to steady yourself, and hallways are typically clear spaces for moving about. If you are comfortable practicing outside, you can walk further. If you stay indoors, make sure you have enough space to walk at least 10 to 12 steps.

1. Position the heel of one foot just in front of the toes of your other foot. Your heel and toes should touch or almost touch.
2. Look straight ahead. Choose a spot ahead of you to focus on.

3. Take a step. Put your heel just in front of the toe of your other foot. Keep your gaze on your focus point to keep you steady and upright.

4. Take another step. Continue stepping, placing the heel of the front foot just in front of the toe of the other foot. Try to keep looking at your focus point. Repeat for 10–12 steps.

Visualize: You are walking on a tightrope, suspended above the ground. Your feet need to stay in a narrow line to remain on the tightrope.

Do you need to make it easier? Start with your feet hip-width apart. Make your first step small so that you narrow the distance, but don't worry about trying to get your feet to touch (this may be too narrow for you to be comfortably upright). Stretch out your arms to the side, to increase your base of support. Or stand close to a wall and hang on as you walk forward, touching the wall without leaning against it.

Are you ready to make it harder? Keep going! Try to complete three to five minutes of heel-toe walking.

Side Bends

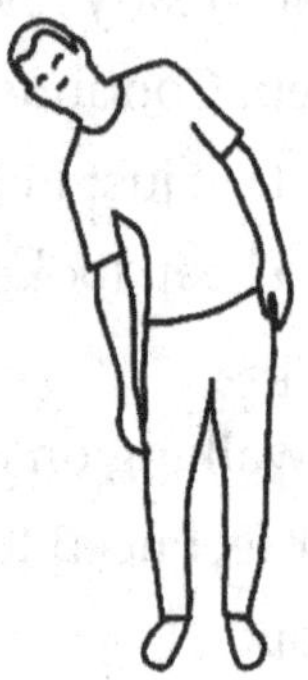

Side bends work the muscles along the sides of your torso, helping to increase your upper body strength and maintain an upright posture.

To start: Stand tall with your feet facing forward, hip-width apart.

1. Place your arms at your sides, fingertips facing down towards the floor.
2. At your waist, lean to your right side with your fingertips reaching towards the floor.
3. Move back to your starting position.
4. Continue bending to the right and up again five to 10 times.

Follow steps 1 to 4 on the left side.

Visualize: You're a teapot wedged between two sheets of glass, tipping over from the waist without leaning forward or back.

Do you need to make it easier? You can sit in a chair to complete the side bends.

Are you ready to make it harder? Add a small can or light weight to the hand on your bending side.

75

Sideways Walking

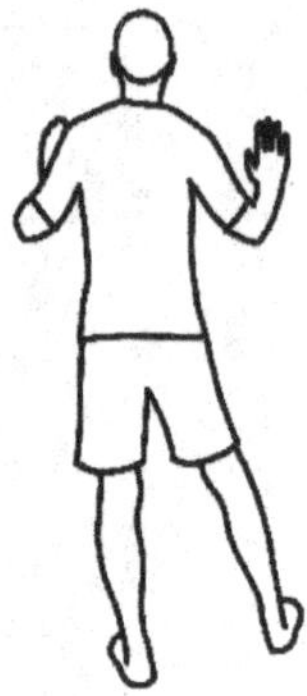

Sideways walking strengthens smaller muscles along the inside and outside of our legs and improves lower-body coordination. Before you do this exercise, check that the space to your right and left is clear of obstacles.

To start: Begin by standing up. Face the wall and place your hands on it as you begin to walk sideways.

1. Foot position: Keep your toes and heels pointed towards the wall. Look down at your feet and make sure both are pointing forwards—sometimes toes like to turn outwards.
2. Left foot: Lift your left foot and move it to the left, then place it back on the ground.
3. Right foot: Lift your right foot and move it closer to your left foot, then place it back on the ground. Continue stepping to the left for five to ten steps. The amount of space you have will dictate how many steps you can take.

4. Change direction: Stay facing the wall to move in the other direction. Lift your right foot and move it to the right, then place it back on the ground.

5. Left foot: Lift your left foot and move it closer to your right foot, then place it back on the ground. Continue stepping to the right for five to ten steps.

Do you need to make it easier? Sit down and take a break before you change direction. Just remember to start at the same place you paused and move the other way.

Are you ready to make it harder? Keep switching directions and aim for five minutes of sideways walking.

High March

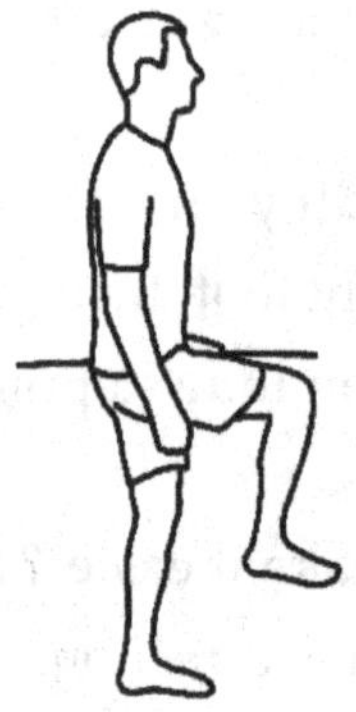

The standing high march is a strength exercise that creates stability on both sides of the body. You are working on your balance at the same time that you are improving core stability. Strong muscles and bones allow us to lift our legs and feet over obstacles, and avoid shuffling when walking, which can lead to falls.

To start: Stand near a wall, counter, or sturdy chair and make sure you can reach it with your hand. Think of a soldier marching in place.

1. Lift: Lift one knee up to hip level and hold it up for three to five seconds.
2. Lower: Use control to lower the leg to the starting position. (Don't use gravity!)
3. Repeat: Repeat Steps 1 and 2 on the other leg.
4. Aim for ten marches, alternating sides with each repetition.

Visualize: Your torso, from just above your hips right up to the top of your head, is frozen in a solid block of ice, and you can only move your legs up and down.

Do you need to make it easier? Start with as many as you can, and work your way up to ten. Sit down and take a break between each repetition. Sit on the edge of a sturdy chair and perform the marches in a seated position.

Are you ready to make it harder? Do a second set of ten marches.

Four-Way Hip Strengthener

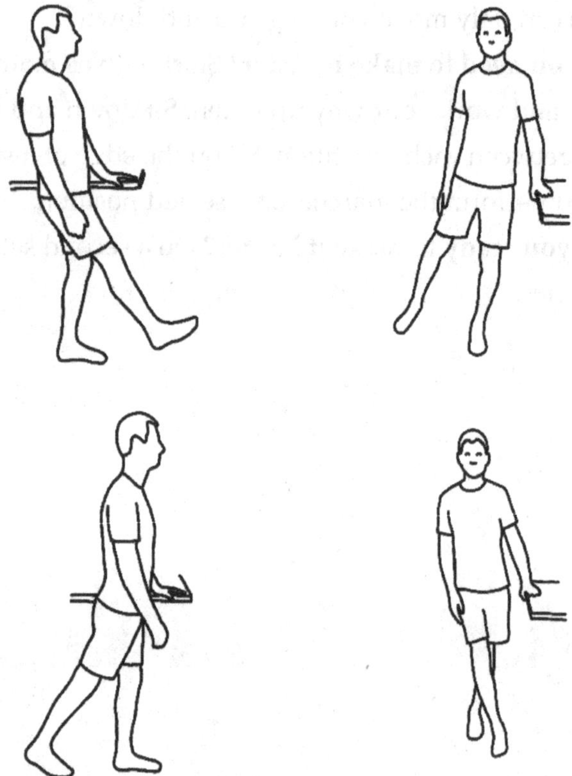

The four-way hip is a strength exercise that helps build stability and flexibility so you can move with ease and avoid injury. You are working on your balance at the same time that you are improving core stability.

To start: Stand near a wall, desk, or sturdy chair and hang on with your right hand. You will move your left leg in four directions, so make sure you won't hit anything as you lift and lower your leg.

1. Forward: Keeping your left leg straight, slowly lift it forward and lower it just as slowly to the

starting position. Don't swing it back and forth; use control to move it.

2. Side: Lift your straight leg out to the side and back to the starting position. Don't lean over to try and lift it higher.

3. Back: Squeeze your bum and lift your leg behind you and back to the starting position. Don't lean forward in an attempt to lift the leg higher.

4. Across: Lift your straight leg across your standing leg and back to the starting position.

5. Repeat: Repeat the entire sequence three to five times on the same leg.

6. Other leg: To repeat on the right leg, move to the other side of the chair and hang on to the chair with your left hand. If you're hanging on to a desk or wall, turn around and hold on with your left hand. Repeat Steps 1 to 5 on your right leg.

Visualize: Your leg is a solid block and you are pushing something heavy with your foot.

Do you want to make it easier? Bend your knees, both on the standing leg and the working leg. Take frequent breaks and sit down to rest.

Are you ready to make it harder? Do 10 repetitions in each direction before you move on to the next position (e.g., lift forward 10 times, then lift to the side 10 times, etc).

APPENDIX A: YOUR MOVEMENT CHECKLIST

Spend time reflecting on how you can add mini movement breaks to your work day. Below you'll find an introductory movement checklist to get you thinking differently about how you work. And I hope it encourages you to sit less and move more.

My Desk

- Move phone just far enough away so I have to stand up to answer it.
- Place documents at the far end of my desk or on another surface.
- Work on engaging more muscles when sitting (aka active sitting).

Nudges*

- Set a timer to get up and move every hour.
- Use my smartphone to set a timer; take that phone and put it on the other side of my office.
- Change my computer screensaver and smartphone screen lock to a message or image that will encourage me to move more.
- Use sticky notes to post reminders to move more.

- Implement mini-movement breaks: 30 seconds every 10 minutes to stand up or even stretch at my desk.

Moving Beyond My Desk

- Send my print jobs to a printer that is farther away from my desk.
- Take the "long cut" when I have to get up from my desk for whatever reason.
- Use a restroom on another floor and take the stairs to and from it.
- Take a SMOKE break. (SMOKE: Sedentary & Movement Optional Kills Early)**

Standing & Waiting

- Get up, stand up. Repeat.
- Work on engaging more muscles when standing (aka active standing).
- Kitchen duty: add movement while waiting for the microwave, kettle, etc.
- Balance on one leg while waiting for the elevator.

Meetings & Interacting with Colleagues

- Volunteer to be the gopher during meetings.
- Implement a standing or walking meeting tradition.
- Walk to a colleague's desk instead of emailing them.

- Recruit co-workers to participate in a "Move More Challenge."

Boss—Do It for the Team

- Walk the talk. Be a movement champion in your office, model movement-based behaviour.
- Send email/text reminders to employees to get up and move, two minutes every hour and 30 seconds every 10 minutes.
- Set policy to have IT implement "farthest" printer settings on employees' computers.
- Set policy to have IT send email reminders to employees, encouraging them to get up and move more.
- Encourage employees to change screensavers to motivational movement images and sayings.
- Implement movement breaks during seated meetings.
- Arrange conference rooms to allow meeting participants to get up and stand without disrupting the flow of the meeting.
- Implement standing or walking meetings.
- Post movement challenges at and in elevators, common areas, meeting rooms.
- Have maintenance paint footprints leading to the stairwells.
- Have maintenance paint faces/eyes on the stairwell doors with speech bubbles, "Will you take the stairs with me?"

***Nudges:** A nudge is simply a way to attract your attention; for instance, putting something at eye level so you notice it. Nudge theory, popularized by behavioural economist Richard Thaler, involves creating small changes in the environment that are designed to change someone's behaviour.[xi] These nudges should be inexpensive and easy to implement, such as leaving fresh fruit on the counter to encourage healthy food choices.

****SMOKE Breaks:** It's still socially acceptable to go for a smoke break at work. And because of indoor no-smoking laws, they have to leave the building to do so. Somehow it is less socially acceptable to leave your desk to take a walk. But we know that incorporating more movement in our lives is not optional. A sedentary lifestyle leads to premature aging and death. We NEED to move more throughout the day.

So tell your boss you're taking a healthy SMOKE break for your body and your mind. And then get up from your desk and move. Go for a walk, stretch your arms up to the sky, twist and turn as you re-energize yourself head to toe. Not everything in our lives needs to be all or nothing. Just because you can't make it to the gym doesn't mean you can't move. Even if you do go to the gym, you should still incorporate those snacks of movement into your daily life. Like pacing, which I'll cover next.

[xi]   Richard H. Thaler and Cass R. Sunstein, *Nudge: Improving Decisions About Health, Wealth, and Happiness*, (New York: Penguin Books, 2008).

REVIEWS AND TESTIMONIALS

"I really enjoyed *Balance and Your Body*! I had fun doing the exercises with my parents (aged 88 and 87). It gets them going, as well as me. It all makes sense—you have to read it and start exercising."

— Teresa

"Balance and Your Body is Amanda's second book especially written for seniors. The message is simple and true: "Move more, stay healthy longer!" The book is well organized and fun to read; the exercises are easy to follow and can be practiced whenever you have some time throughout the day (or sleepless night). No gym or equipment required!"

— An enthusiastic senior

"Her new book, *Balance and Your Body*, is very clear and easy to read. She explains why we need to move and the different aspects of balance. The exercises are simple and drawings help understand them. Not at all overwhelming to do the exercises. A very helpful book for any senior concerned about maintaining their independence. Essential for seniors to stay independent. Well done!"

— Amazon customer

"As a teacher and musician, I suffer from several repetitive strain injuries and back problems related to performance. *Move More, Your Life Depends On It* is a huge wake up call for so many of us who live our lives behind a computer and think there isn't any opportunity in our daily routine to exercise. Amanda's book showed me that there are countless opportunities throughout each day to exercise and reduce some of the chronic pain I experience just by doing my daily tasks. I highly recommend it for anyone in any industry."

— Danielle Allard, singer/songwriter

"*Move More, Your Life Depends On It* contains simple and powerful tips I have incorporated into my daily life. This book ranks as one of my favorites. The information is inspiring, timeless, well-organized, and an easy read. Amanda does a great job sharing her knowledge in a fun way."

— Fabiana Meredith, co-founder Qi

"Today while in four hours of meetings I got up and moved around…[I] even walked backwards to the door to excuse myself! Thank you for the tips...already making changes in my day!"

— *Move More* workshop participant

"Amanda, thank you so much for coming to talk to us at Retire-At-Home Services. Our jobs are demanding and require the utmost attention throughout our shifts. Many of our staff have continual neck and back pain due to the time they spend sitting & answering phones and typing. I really am thankful that you sent an important message to keep moving throughout our days. The simple tips and stretches you provided are invaluable to our staff! I believe every office would benefit from Amanda's presentation. Thanks again!"

— Catherine Bennett, Retire-At-Home

ABOUT THE AUTHOR

Amanda Sterczyk is an author and personal trainer based in Ottawa, Canada. In 2016, she founded The Move More Institute™, an initiative to promote healthy active living and teach individuals how to sneak "exercise" into their daily lives. Her slogan is "Move more, feel better." Amanda holds a Master's degree in social psychology from Carleton University. *Sweat-Free Exercises for the Office* is her eighth book.

You can connect with Amanda online by visiting her website: http://www.amandasterczyk.com. "Add Movement at Work" is now available as a free course on Thinkific.